NATURAL
Perfumes

SIMPLE AROMATHERAPY RECIPES

Mindy Green

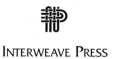

INTERWEAVE PRESS

The contents of this book are not intended as a substitute for medical treatment, nor should they be used as such. Consult your physician or other health-care practitioner in all matters affecting your health, and carefully follow the advice you receive.

Natural Perfumes
by Mindy Green

Editor, Susan Clotfelter
Cover design, Bren Frisch
Photography, Joe Coca
Illustration, Ann Sabin Swanson
Book design, Dean Howes

Text copyright, © 1999, Mindy Green

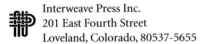 Interweave Press Inc.
201 East Fourth Street
Loveland, Colorado, 80537-5655

Printed in China by Midas

Library of Congress Cataloging-in-Publication Data
Green, Mindy.
    Natural perfumes : simple aromatherapy recipes / by Mindy Green.
       p.   cm.
    Includes bibliographical references.
    ISBN 1-883010-62-4
    1. Perfumes.I. Title.
TP 983.G671999
668'.542–dc21   99-24391
                                             CIP

First Printing: 7.5M:599:CC

To all those willing to

explore their creativity

through nature

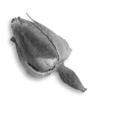
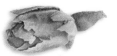

Contents

Invitation

What is more mysterious than a fragrance floating on the air, just within perception, but just beyond description? Although the sense of smell affects us in fundamental ways, it often thwarts our efforts to describe it. Scent can conjure feelings that stir the depths of the soul. But because this ability is invisible, it seems both obscure and all the more powerful.

Scent can delight and repel, attract and repulse. It can evoke happy or melancholy memories, influence buying behavior, and signal sexual readiness. More recently, researchers are discovering that essential oils, the concentrated liquid fragrances of plants, can not only affect mood, but stimulate physical reactions as well. In other words, scent heals. How delightful to discover that something so luxurious for the soul also benefits the body.

For myself, creating fragrances from natural plant essences has been a spiritual journey. Early on, I found myself wondering about the complex mechanisms of plants. How does the smell get in there? How do plants know that they are supposed to produce a certain color flower, or attract a particular insect for pollination, or make a specific chemical constituent? How is it that a tree being attacked by insects knows to create a special chemical to repel them, or signal to other trees, miles away, to prepare their own chemicals for an imminent attack? How does a flower know to change color after pollination? How are plants and their fragrances able to excite emotion or influence healing?

Such mysteries remind me daily why I chose to make my living with herbs more than twenty-seven years ago. For me, creating perfumes from natural plant essences is an amazing thrill. I hope that after learning about natural perfumes through this book, you will find your own exciting path to discovering something new about nature and fragrance.

Other than olfactory adventure — a superb reason in itself — why should you want to make your own perfume and aromatherapy products? There are several reasons. When you buy a commercial perfume, you pay for high advertising budgets and executive salaries. When you see how much a blend of alcohol, water, and the merest smidge of actual essential oils costs, you'll understand that those dollars can purchase a lot more satisfaction when you blend your own fragrances. In addition, scent preference is an extremely personal matter. I have taught aromatherapy classes where some people must leave the room when I pass a sample of rose or lavender. Those same students adore the smells of tea tree and thyme. There is no accounting for taste. Only you will ever know which scents you like best, and which ones inspire, relax, or invigorate you. When you make your own scents, you can choose the elements to combine.

There is no doubt in my mind that once you're comfortable with the art of aromatic blending, you will never purchase synthetic perfumes again. You'll be pleasantly surprised when total strangers ask where they can purchase the scent you are wearing; you'll have the joy of saying that you created this unique fragrance yourself. This really does happen! Early one Saturday morning, I had a postal worker discuss with me at length the sickening chemical fragrances to which working with the public exposed her. She went on to say she liked my perfume and asked what I was wearing. Nothing, I thought, because I hadn't had time to shower yet. I couldn't smell a thing. Then I remembered the perfume I had worn the previous night to go out dancing. Heavy with base notes, it still lingered, though I had used it quite sparingly.

Perhaps the most compelling reason to make your own natural perfumes is to connect to nature, to be reminded of a world full of life-force, to be aflame with a desire to experience pleasure. Natural perfumes connect us at a soul level to the earth and to our own spirituality. They are a link between us and the greater cosmos. They tell us we are part of a greater whole, and always one with the flowers.

— *Mindy Green*

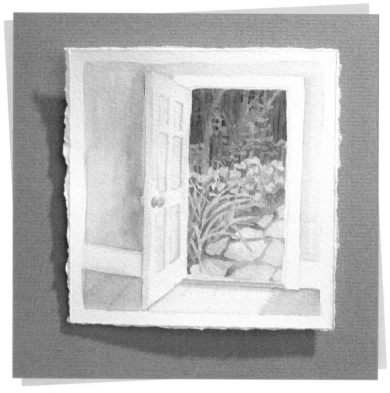

"*Smell is a potent wizard that transports us across thousands of miles . . .*"

— Helen Keller

The Science and Allure of Scent

Breath is our most direct communication with nature. It is *prana,* life. We monitor the air around us with every breath we take, the scent of violets transporting us to a field of flowers, the smell of smoke alerting us to danger. Although we now use reason to find food, shelter, and a mate, our brain's primitive link between smell and reaction remains. The aroma of food can trigger hunger, even though you may not be aware you haven't eaten in hours. It will even start the involuntary flow of digestive juices. The sense of smell is a communication system, though we are not always aware of the messages we are sending or receiving.

Smell was our first sense as we evolved. The small lump of olfactory tissue atop the nerve cord eventually developed into a brain. The two halves of the brain began as bumps on the olfactory stalks. Some scientists theorize that we are able to think at all because first we *smelled.* The olfactory nerve is the first cranial nerve. Olfactory neurons are the only ones in the body that regenerate themselves, doing so about every thirty days. This is a clue to the biological importance of smell in the survival of species. Smell is 10,000 times more sensitive than the other senses. The tongue tastes only sweet, sour, salt, and bitter; all other shades of difference, odor creates. (We have all experienced what a lack of this sense does to our world during a cold—we can't taste a thing.)

Smell is also the only sense whose receptor nerve endings are in direct contact with the outside world. The olfactory membrane, or the pathway from the nose to the brain, is exposed to the environment. Each little nerve cell in it acts as a tiny branch of the brain; for all intents and purposes, the brain extends directly to the nose. Sight, sound, and the other senses are processed via the thalamus and the cerebral cortex—the left side, or thinking part of the brain. Smell, however, is processed via the brain's right side, the area that governs emotion and creativity. Smell causes us to respond non-rationally—before we can think.

Scientists have a number of theories on how we recognize odor, but the most popular is that scent molecules have shapes that match specific receptor sites, allowing us to distinguish between odors. When we inhale odor molecules, they bind to one of the human body's 20 million olfactory epithelium cells, or receptors, in the olfactory membrane. Next, a message is fired to the olfactory bulb, whose neurons transmit this message to the limbic system, the seat of emotion and memory. The limbic system activates the hypothalamus. The pituitary, on cue from the hypothalamus, releases chemical messages into the bloodstream, activating hormones and regulating body functions. Depending on the chemistry of the odor molecules, this process has the ability to influence sex drive, appetite, body temperature, insulin production, stress levels, and metabolism, as well as affect thoughts and emotions. Mood actually does affect odor. The production of adrenaline changes your smell. Some animals *can* detect fear, because it has an odor.

Studies show that odors can change brain wave activity. An electroencephalogram, or electronic reading of brain waves, demonstrates that smelling lavender stimulates alpha waves in the brain, resulting in relaxation. The scent of jasmine, on the other hand, stimulates beta waves, making a person feel awake and alert.

PHEROMONES, SEX, AND FRAGRANCE

One of the most intriguing areas of scent research probes how aromas can trigger emotional and sexual reactions. Smell and sensuality have always had a strong link. We may wax poetic about visual attraction, but often, it is actually odor that is the initiating factor in sexual attraction. In one survey conducted in Wales, 71 percent of both men and women said smell was the biggest factor in sexual attraction.

So what's behind the power of scent in the mating dance? Pheromones may have paved the way. These chemical substances are produced by one individual and affect the physiological, sexual responses of another—usually, the intended mate or mates. The word pheromone was coined in 1959, from the Greek "pherein," to carry, and "hormon," to excite, or to transfer excitement. Scientists believe that pheromones are by-products of reproductive hormones to which they are chemically similar. Humans start secreting pheromones at puberty, giving a unique scent to perspiration, part of the subtle signal that attracts the opposite sex. This makes perfect evolutionary sense; there is no reason to signal reproductive readiness before it occurs.

Fragrance manufacturers, hoping to cash in on this concept, sometimes base fragrances (or just their marketing appeals) on pheromonal attraction. Historically, aphrodisiac scents relied on animal-derived fragrances such as musk, civet and castoreum, from anal or sex glands of the musk deer, civet cat, and beaver, respectively. By the Elizabethan era the reputed aphrodisiac powers of these scents were well-known.

On the other hand, at full strength these smells are not very pleasant. But used correctly, in nearly undetectable amounts, they can produce the right results. I actually like the smell of skunk—but only from many miles away. This is a good example of the importance of proportion and odor intensity, which are discussed in the chapters about blending and essential oils.

Some of what you might think are human pheromonal odors are often considered unpleasant. In fact, we are encouraged to buy products—underarm deodorants and others—precisely to hide these odors. But keep in mind that sweat only develops an odor when it has time to react with bacteria. Fresh perspiration, or the aroma of freshly showered skin, are very different smells.

There are fragrant chemicals found in essential oils that can mimic or enhance our own pheromones.

There are fragrant chemicals found in essential oils that can mimic or enhance our own pheromones, or at least trigger hormones that may influence pheromone production. For instance, sandalwood oil is said to contain chemicals similar to androgen-like hormones; clary sage and fennel oils contain phytosterols that promote human hormonal activity; and ambrette seed oil is a plant substitute for animal musk. Other famous "aphrodisiac" scents include lavender, rose, jasmine, and ylang ylang. One study by Dr. Alan Hirsch, director of the Smell and Taste Research and Treatment Center in Chicago, showed that the odor of lavender essential oil increased penile blood flow.

We probably think of flowers as being aphrodisiacs because they are, in fact, the sex organs of plants. In full bloom, they advertise their desire to be pollinated. No wonder flowers attract us. No wonder we wear their scents to attract others.

Consumers and Scent

When you shop for shampoo, do you twist off the cap to find out what it smells like? Probably. Recent studies illustrate how odors can manipulate buying behavior. We don't need to be aware of a fragrance for it to affect us. Among the many studies Dr. Hirsch has conducted on the power of scent, one shows that consumers are willing to spend more for athletic shoes when the sales environment is scented, even though the scent was not strong enough for them to consciously notice. In another study at a Las Vegas casino, a special odor was piped into a separate area. Gamblers spent 40 percent more in that area. In another study, a group of participants reported that a scented brand of paint went on smoother and covered better than an identical, unscented brand. A similar study found the same result with hosiery. Whatever effect you are trying to achieve with scent, this research suggests that using it subtly may be your best strategy.

We don't need to be aware of a fragrance for it to affect us.

The Basics of Aromatherapy

Aromatherapy is the use of pure essential oils to enhance health, beauty and psychological well-being. French chemist René-Maurice Gattefossé coined the term in 1928. After an accidental burn in his laboratory, he plunged his hand into the nearest container of liquid. It happened to be lavender oil. Gattefossé noticed that the oil stopped the pain and helped his skin heal quickly without scarring. Thus began his inquiry into the field of aromatic chemistry. Gattefossé was one of the first to proclaim that essential oils in their whole form work better than their synthetic counterparts or isolated constituents.

Essential oils are absorbed into the body through the skin or by inhalation. The skin absorbs essential oils readily because their molecules are extremely small, and because they are lipid soluble, meaning they are readily taken up by the sebum that our skin produces. Once essential oils have penetrated the skin, they can enter the capillaries, lymphatic vessels and nerve cells that run through the lower layer of skin cells.

Inhaled essential oil components enter the bloodstream through the lungs. But first, they have their most profound effect during their journey through the olfactory system. Once the olfactory cell receptors detect an odor, they alert the area of the brain that processes odor, known as the limbic system. This area controls memory and emotion, sex drive, fight-or-flight mechanism, and other instinctual processes. Smelling essential oils can stimulate neurotransmitters to release body chemicals that spur a host of different reactions.

WHAT ARE ESSENTIAL OILS?

Essential oils come from plants. Often, they contain the components that give healing herbs their medicinal qualities. A

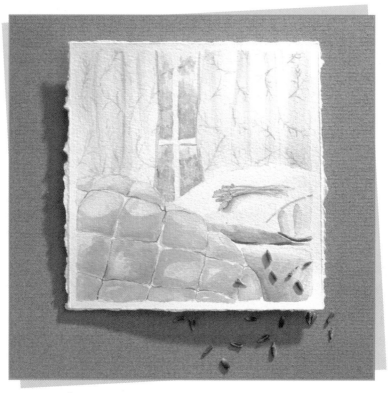

"*Look in the perfumes of flowers and
of nature for peace of mind
and joy of life.*"

— *Wang Wei*

single plant can contain 350 or more individual chemical constituents with a wide range of effects, such as fighting bacteria, inhibiting viruses, calming cramps, or soothing digestion. Produced in tiny sacs or canals within plant cells, essential oils can occur in any plant part: seeds (carrot and coriander), flowers (rose and chamomile), leaves (geranium and rosemary), needles (fir and pine), roots (vetiver and valerian), rhizomes (ginger), wood (cinnamon and cedar), and resins (frankincense and myrrh). Some plants have essential oils in more than one part, such as the orange, which produces petitgrain oil in the leaves, neroli oil in the blossoms, and orange oil in the peel.

Essential oils usually perform vital functions within the plant itself. Their odors may attract pollinators or provide protection from predators tempted to nibble young branches. The evaporation of essential oils from the surfaces of some leaves protects the plant from fungus or yeast organisms that can otherwise set up housekeeping on the plant.

HOW ESSENTIAL OILS ARE MADE

Perfumers extract essential oils from plants by several means, mostly distillation. When the plant parts—be they roots, seeds, leaves, or flowers—are exposed to heat, the oil-containing cellular sacs burst. The oils evaporate with the steam, which is then recondensed. Essential oils are not water soluble, so they usually float, making them easy to capture.

Heat, however, destroys the odors of some flowers—for example, jasmine. For such plants, essential oils are extracted by solvents. The flowers are submerged in hexane, petroleum ether, or another solvent with a low boiling point. After agitation, perfumers remove the solvent under pressure, producing a solid substance called a concrete. Alcohol is added and agitated to dissolve plant waxes, then the alcohol and suspended wax also are removed. The resulting product is called an absolute. Technically speaking, absolutes are not essential oils, although they do contain the plant's fragrance. They are used mainly in the perfume industry because processing without heat yields a product truer to the odor of the plant. Some fragrances are available in either absolute or essential oil. Rose is a good example, but other absolutes less commonly used in aromatherapy are clary sage, lavender, and rosemary. Some aromatherapists avoid absolutes altogether because they're concerned about solvent residues in the final extract, or because they don't wish to support the use of these solvents. Others feel that absolutes have greater healing potential because the processing method leaves a wider range of chemical constituents in the extract. The controversy rages on. For purposes of fragrance blending, absolutes offer more variety, since distilled essential oils of many rare flowers and other plants are unavailable. However, such absolutes are expensive and hard to find, so we won't discuss them in depth.

Enfleurage is one of the oldest methods of extraction, similar in process to solvent extraction, but using animal fats. It is not often done these days, because it is time-consuming and labor-intensive. Nonetheless, you may occasionally come across an enfleurage of tuberose or jasmine.

Another method of extraction, cold expression (sometimes called scarification) is used solely for citrus peels. The oil is literally squeezed from the peel. Some citrus essential oils, such as lime oil, may also be distilled.

Carbon dioxide extraction is the newest method. Because of equipment costs, it is expensive, but produces a superior scent. No solvents are used, so it is ecologically sound. And no heat is used, so no healing or fragrance components are destroyed. The essential oils most often extracted this way are spices such as ginger, clove, and nutmeg. These essences are used by the food and flavoring industry but are also sold by some aromatherapy companies. They are favorites of mine for their scent and purity, but they are not widely available.

Essential oils are highly concentrated substances. For example, it takes thirty to sixty roses to make one drop of rose essential oil.

Essential oils are highly concentrated substances. For example, it takes thirty to sixty roses to make one drop of rose essential oil. To make a pound of essential oil, it takes twenty pounds of clove buds, thirty to fifty pounds of eucalyptus leaves, 150 pounds of lavender flowers, and 2,000 to 3,000 pounds of rose petals.

NATURAL VS. SYNTHETIC OILS

Aromatherapists believe that plant-derived essential oils act differently than synthetic simulations. Obviously, natural essential oils come from plants and synthetics are produced in a laboratory. Sometimes synthetic fragrances start with natural oils, such as turpentine, but just as often the starting oil is petroleum-based. Even when the chemical structure of a component—for example, geraniol from scented geraniums—is the same whether it comes from natural or synthetic sources, aromatherapists argue that the natural essential oil contains an unquantifiable "life force." Studies do show that many natural oils have more beneficial effects than their synthetic rivals. Also, many aromatherapists believe that natural essential oils provoke fewer allergic reactions. It's my theory that our bodies have a biological familiarity with the natural oils.

Most commercial perfumes produced today are a combination of many synthetic ingredients and a few natural oils. The American perfume industry uses only about 20 percent natural essential oils. It may surprise you to learn that most of the products we encounter daily are synthetically perfumed, including plastics, fabrics, automobile interiors, shampoos, children's toys, carpet, laundry detergents and other household cleaners, cosmetics, even medicines. We are all bombarded daily with artificial fragrances that are difficult to avoid. Why further burden our bodies with synthetic perfumes, especially when natural ones are now so easy to obtain?

Natural perfumery uses pure botanical essences. It recognizes that each person has his or her own unique and potentially beautiful scent, and that perfume is meant to enhance, indulge and accentuate each individual odor-print. Natural perfumes are not synthetic, chemical smells meant to cover up odors, but our planet's primal and genuine essences, a part of the transactions of nature. They are an expression of the best that scent can be.

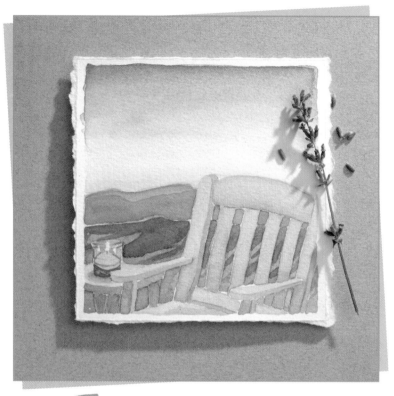

*"The sense of smell is the
sense of the imagination."*

—Jean-Jacques Rousseau

Blending Fundamentals

romatic blending can be challenging and intimidating to the beginning natural perfume enthusiast. But with a basic understanding of some elementary principles and a bit of imagination, anyone can create wonderful and distinctive perfume blends. Endless pleasures await you!

First, however, a word about safety. Essential oils, the tools of natural perfumery, are very concentrated substances. *Never use them undiluted on the skin.* To make the preparations in this book, you will always dilute essential oil blends in what is called a carrier oil, such as almond, jojoba or sesame oil.

It is also very important that the oils be pure plant extracts, not synthetic fragrance oils. Read labels carefully, ask your supplier questions, and look for the Latin names of plants to make sure that you're purchasing the oil that you desire. Ideally, a label will specify the following: the common name and Latin binomial of the plant used, the plant *parts* used, the extraction process, the plant's country of origin, and how the plant was grown—certified organic, cultivated or wildcrafted, etc. (Few companies may offer all that information on a small bottle, but most are happy to share it if you contact them.)

You must also choose the oils you use with careful regard to skin sensitivity—your own or any other people for whom you are blending a product. Consider the proportion of essential oils to carrier oils that you use, and make weaker dilutions for children, those who are pregnant or nursing, or for anyone who is highly allergic. See the Forty Fragrant Oils chapter for further safety guidelines for individual oils.

When making a perfume blend, consider its purpose. If you are making a scent for therapeutic or cosmetic use, do some further research into the medicinal qualities of the oils you're considering. While this book focuses on blending for fun and fragrance, it also includes brief information on how aromatherapists use each oil for physical and emotional healing. The most important consideration is whether you like the scent, but even the simplest perfume blends can have some therapeutic qualities; the very same oils go into medicinal and cosmetic products. Becoming familiar with the various properties of the oils will ensure that you create a balanced blend with staying power and healing power.

While there are no hard and fast rules for creating your own blend, following a few safety precautions and guidelines about proportion will help you create delightful fragrances with greater success and less practice.

FRAGRANCE NOTES

Top, middle, and base notes are terms that perfumers use to describe scents. They are based on the evaporation rate of essential oils. Most base notes are thick, oily, dark, viscous liquids with a slow evaporation rate. Top notes tend to be thin, runny, and often clear; they evaporate quickly. When you smell a particular fragrance, the top notes are the ones you notice first.

Some single essential oils are so complex they may actually fit into two or even all three categories, depending on the other oils in the blend. For example, in some recipes, rose or clary sage will act as middle notes, while in others they will function as base notes. Angelica and peppermint also cross categories; they can be top or middle notes.

Top Notes

Top notes, the fastest evaporating oils, are sometimes referred to as head or peak notes. In a perfume blend, these ephemeral fragrances hit the nose first, then quickly dissipate. They tend to be light, fresh, sharp, and penetrating. They can last on the body as long as thirty minutes, but may diffuse more quickly. They can make up five to twenty percent of your blend.

Therapeutically, the actions of top notes are used to stimulate and uplift the spirit. Examples include most citrus oils, fruit peels, and lemongrass. Citrus top notes have a comparatively short shelf life. They keep well for about one year without refrigeration. Large quantities of citrus oils are best kept refrigerated.

Middle Notes

Middle notes, also called bouquet or heart notes, should be the main body of a blend. They round it out, creating soothing, softer tones or harmonizing top and base notes. They last as long as three hours after application, and can make up 50 to 80 percent of a blend.

Therapeutically, middle notes are usually essential oils that are thought to have harmonizing and balancing actions. This category includes chamomile, geranium, and lavender. Most middle notes will keep for five years or more if stored away from heat and light (for more about storing fragrances, see the section on shelf life on page 26)

Base Notes

Sometimes referred to as dry or fond notes, base notes provide a deep, warm, sensuous quality. They give your blend tenacity. They often function as fixatives, holding back the evaporation of top notes. Use them rather sparingly, as they often are not very pleasant when used alone or full strength. In proper proportion, however, they can add great depth and intensity to a blend. By three to four hours after application, most of the lingering odor of a scent will be the base note. These oils will usually make up 5 to 10 percent of the total blend, but if a base note is pleasing, you can use up to 20 percent.

Aromatherapists use sedating base notes to relieve anxiety, stress, impatience, and insomnia. Most woods, resins, and roots are base notes; they tend to be among the most expensive essential oils. Some of the more pleasing base notes include cedar, sandalwood, frankincense, vanilla, and jasmine. Base notes that you may choose to use more sparingly include spikenard, vetiver, and patchouli. Base notes have the longest shelf life; they actually improve with age. A twenty-year-old patchouli will soften in fragrance, thicken in viscosity, and darken in color.

If you want to create an uplifting blend for depression, it may be top note heavy. If you fancy something deep, sultry, earthy, and mysterious, it may be heavy with base notes. Be experimental and creative; you're doing this for fun! There are no right or wrong fragrances. If you like it, you've done it correctly.

STARTING FROM SCRATCH

Here's how a basic blending session begins. Before you start, you'll want to finish this chapter so you'll be familiar with the whole process. I recommend continuing reading at least through Two Beginning Blending Lessons before purchasing your materials.

Gather Your Equipment

To begin, make a list of the oils you consider appropriate or the ones you'd like to experiment with. Then trim it down to four or five, based on the note categories, possible duplication, oil availability or expense. Consider what kind of scented products you'd like to make from your essential oil blend. If you only wish to make perfume, you'll need jojoba oil and bottles to hold your blend. If you wish to make splashes, colognes, or spritzes, you'll need grain alcohol, distilled water, and other additional materials. You'll want strips of blotter paper or other absorbent paper for testing your scents; you can run out of pulse points on your arm pretty quickly.

The sources listed in the Resource Directory can help you find essential oils and carrier oils by mail order if you can't obtain them in your area.

Create Your Mood

Different seasons or times of day may inspire different scents. A bright summer day or an early morning activity may bring to mind a light fresh fragrance with a predominant top note to invigorate and refresh. At night or in the winter months, a heavier, base note perfume that is deep and sensuous may be more inspiring. Representational perfumes are ones that imitate a known substance: a flower, the scent of leather, or a fine tea blend. Abstract perfumes attempt to create a feeling or celebrate an occasion such as a hot summer day, the moment before a thunderstorm, a picnic celebration, or Christmas morning. Give some thought to what sort of blend you would like to create. Let it roll through your psyche and thoughts, conjuring adventurous days or romantic nights.

As you prepare to create your blend, take a moment to consider its purpose. Clear intent is important; I believe it adds its own power to your formula. You may find it useful to have a moment of silence in a special place while you reflect on your intended outcome.

Ready, Set, Sniff

Now you are ready to blend. This can be an intimidating part of the process, as one drop too much can throw off the whole balance. Begin working out your blend on paper, listing the oils and their approximate proportions. It is important to keep detailed notes of your process, so that you can learn from mistakes and duplicate successes.

Smell each of your intended oils. Open the bottles one by one and imagine in your mind how they will blend with each other. You can hold the bottle caps to your nose in differing combinations, or better yet, use strips of labeled blotter paper or cut-up coffee filters. Just put a dab of oil on each and wave different combinations of them under your nose.

Ultimately, a fragrance must be tested on the skin to give a true perspective of how it will affect you and those around you. What smells good in a bottle may smell very differently on the body. To test the oils on your skin, dip a toothpick into the oil and barely touch it to your inner wrist. Let the oil warm and breathe for a moment, then sniff. Now try layering the other possible components of your blend on top; this will give you a good idea of how particular essential oils interact with your skin and with each other. Notice that with this step, you're violating the cardinal aromatherapy rule about not applying undiluted oils to your skin. That's why you want to use tiny quantities and pay careful attention; if you know you have any allergies or sensitivi-

With some experience, you'll be able to predict with some accuracy how scents change on your body.

ties, avoid those oils, or dilute a very small amount for testing purposes. With some experience, you'll be able to predict with some accuracy how scents change on your body.

Now you're ready to begin combining oils in a bottle. If you're not certain about the proportion, begin with one drop of each oil, and build, sniffing as you go after each addition. You will find that one ingredient may only require one drop while others need ten, fifteen, or more. Keep notes! The blend will change with each addition.

If your sniffer gets overwhelmed, leave the blending for an hour or a day, and then return to it. Olfactory exhaustion, or smell fatigue, occurs after some time, usually ten to thirty minutes depending on the fragrances, room ventilation, or personal sensitivity. A professional perfumer, or "nose," as they are called, works for fifteen minutes on and fifteen minutes off, to keep a fresh "nasal palate." Sniffing fresh ground coffee or going outdoors for some fresh air can help reset your nose.

BASIC BLENDING EQUIPMENT

Blending surface: a large synthetic cutting board or any surface (except wood); covered with oilcloth, waxed paper, or an old towel that will absorb spilled oils

Essential oils, preferably each with its own dropper

Small, preferably dark, glass bottles to hold blends

Additional eyedroppers if needed

Small bottle of grain alcohol with which to clean eyedroppers (just swish, squeeze, and squirt droppers between dispensing oils, then wipe them with a tissue)

Strips of blotter paper

Carrier oils or grain alcohol/water mixture for eau de colognes, splashes

Clean, empty spray bottles for spritzes and splashes

Fresh ground coffee to refresh your nose

Source of fresh air — fan or nearby window

Inspirational music

When you are making notes about your blend, it is helpful to have some descriptive odor terminology to precisely convey what you are noticing. Scent is notoriously difficult to describe. Terms relating to foods or wine are often used, as are shapes, temperatures or even inanimate objects. I sometimes describe synthetic smells as a spike-through-the-forehead odor, or smelling of aluminum foil; though neither of these has an odor, it does evoke an image. Think about it. Does your fragrance feel round, smooth or sharp? Is it voluminous, heavy, or airy? Is it tight, steady, sparse, or scattered? Is it warm and soft or cool and crisp? Assertive or modest? Do you need to bring it down with base notes, elevate it with top notes, or plump it up with middle notes? Where do you feel it in your body—your head, heart or solar plexus? Is it broad or narrow, high-pitched or deep, vigorous or languorous? Is it mossy, green, floral, earthy, woody, or citrusy? Does it remind you of hay, roots, fruit, or nuts? What type of personality would it appeal to: someone flamboyant and outgoing or demure and shy?

It may take a little practice, but soon it will be easy to take charge of your blend and steer it in just the right direction as it develops.

BLENDING SUBTLETIES

Understanding the diffusiveness and volatility of a particular oil is important for constructing a blend. Some essential oils have a much higher odor intensity than others, and much less of a particular oil may be needed to provide equal scent representation in your final outcome. For instance, if you want to make a simple blend of lavender and chamomile, and you wish each scent to be equally represented, you will need only one drop of chamomile to about five drops of lavender. Other essential oils with a high odor intensity include spikenard, patchouli, vetiver, lemongrass and cinnamon, to name a few. The Forty Fragrant Oils chapter contains information about each oil's intensity.

Blends can be made with four different oils and total only ten drops, or more oils and much higher quantities. The quantity you make is up to you. In making a perfume blend, there are no rules for proportion other the level of concentration. I recommend up to half essential oil blend and half carrier oil. However, if you are making your blend into a massage oil, which is applied to the skin in higher quantities, use only about two percent essential oils, or ten to twelve drops total of essential oil blend to each fluid ounce of carrier oil. Using the example of lavender and chamomile again, a simple massage oil would contain 2 to 3 drops of chamomile, 9 drops of lavender, and one fluid ounce of carrier oil.

Always mix essential oils before adding a carrier oil. The essential oils need to "marry" before they are diluted. Hold your blend in your hands and shake or roll it back and forth. Affirm its purpose and intent; keep in mind the person for whom the blend is made. This may well be the most important step in your ritual of blending a natural perfume. I believe that it adds a powerful human energy, positively charging your blend.

Aging

Once made, perfume concentrates—the undiluted essential oil blends—may be aged for several weeks to several months or longer. Aging allows the single essential oils to continue marrying and eventually emerge as a unique cohesive blend with an eloquent character. Your blend will mellow over time, acquiring smoothness and expressiveness. When aged, it should have a full-bodied character; it should not appear "thin" or "tinny." In a carefully constructed perfume blend, top, middle and base notes will unfold distinctly, allowing the blend to deliver all the richness of its complexity.

Shelf Life

If you prefer, you may store your essential oil blends as concentrates, adding no carriers until you are ready to use them as fragrances, bath oil, room spray, etc. Once a blend with a carrier, you should use up the resulting product within six months. Shelf life depends, in part, on the carrier used and environmental conditions. All essential oils, whether in blends or single notes, should be kept away from heat and light. An undiluted blend, heavy on base notes, will improve with age if stored properly, even for several years.

Carriers for Perfume Blends

Jojoba is the carrier oil of choice for natural perfumes. Chemically, it is a wax, not an oil, so it will not go rancid. It is also my favorite choice for skin care products. Jojoba oil is non-comedogenic, meaning it won't plug pores, so it works well for any product to be used on the face. Vitamin E oil, added to products in small quantities, is an excellent antioxidant and natural preservative. The contents of one 400-IU capsule in one ounce of a cosmetic blend, or the contents of two capsules in four ounces of a massage oil, is sufficient. Massage, body, or bath oils may be made with other vegetable oils such as almond, apricot, hazelnut, sunflower, olive, etc.

Distilled water may be used as a carrier if you want to make a light mist suitable for spritzing your body, bedroom sheets, or other linens. (Tap water can also be used, but the spritz will have a shorter life) Essential oils will separate from the water, so shake your spray bottle well before firing away.

Pure grain alcohol (not rubbing alcohol) works well for perfume blends with resinous essential oils that are not readily soluble in jojoba oil. For a cologne or body splash, a combination of alcohol and water is appropriate. The alcohol evaporates quickly, contributing a cooling effect. In the commercial fragrance industry, the only difference between a cologne, eau de toilette, and perfume is the proportion of alcohol/water blend to essential or fragrance oil.

Wearing Your Perfume

Ideally, oils should be applied to the skin to mix with your own body oils, slowing the evaporation rate of the fragrance and creating a scent that is unique on you. The classic application areas are behind the ears, at the throat, or the pulse points, the wrists, inner arms, even behind the knees. These pulse points are where the heat of the body is closest to the skin, giving greater impact to your fragrance. I sometimes put fragrance in my hair, as some suggest that the proteins in hair hold the scent effectively.

ABOUT CARRIER OILS

Here is a brief list of the oils I recommend for aromatherapy uses. Be sure to obtain high-quality, fresh, cold-pressed nut oils, or extra virgin olive oils, and store them out of heat. In fact, all vegetable oils are best stored in the refrigerator.

Use	Oil	Properties
Perfumes and facial care	Jojoba	Holds scent well, won't clog pores; won't spoil; absorbs quickly into skin
Body oils	Olive	Absorbs quickly into skin, good for use as an after-bath oil; readily available; inexpensive
Body or massage oil	Sesame	Stays on skin a bit longer; good for those who are allergic to nut oils or dislike olive
Massage oils	Almond	High in Vitamin E
	Apricot kernel	Holds scent well, good shelf life
	Sunflower	Readily available; inexpensive

However, I highly recommend that you wear your perfume blend on an area of your body that won't be exposed to sunlight. Some natural fragrance ingredients, especially the citrus oils, can cause sun sensitivity from ultraviolet rays. This photosensitization causes increased melanin production in the skin, resulting in potentially serious sunburn or pigmentation problems. These oils can also speed the tanning process—not a good thing, because tanning is an aging process. I suggest applying perfume to the nape of the neck, if your hair is long enough to cover it. If you are highly sensitive you can wear your blend on your clothing, but some essential oils may stain. Also, your blend won't "progress," or blend with your own body's scent, as well, nor last as long.

Oily skin will hold a scent longer than dry skin, so it may not need as much on initial application. Temperature, altitude, and humidity will also affect the development of your fragrance. Scent intensifies in a warm, humid climate, because odor molecules evaporate less readily in moist air. Consider using lighter notes if your environment is warm and humid. In a dry or cool climate, reapply scent more often or use heavier scents. The thin air at high altitudes also reduces a fragrance's staying power.

Less Is More

Sometimes it helps to layer a fragrance. After a shower, start with a light splash or mist over the entire body. Then dab pulse points with the same fragrance in perfume strength. If you choose to apply fragrance lightly, do so low on the body, as scent rises and the fragrance will seem to last longer as it wafts upward.

Though the use of perfume can add to your feeling of well-being, you should never wear too much! It is always better to be understated. Your fragrance "aura" should not extend beyond arm's length. It should remain a personal and subtle message, enticing those around you to come closer, to be drawn into your circle of scent. A perfume blend is successfully worn if it uplifts the wearer, but is not overbearing. It must be appropriate to the surroundings, have staying power, unfold evenly, and be dermatologically safe. Above all, your blend should exhibit vigor and diffusion while maintaining a sense of delicate clarity and character.

PROPORTIONS FOR FRAGRANCE PRODUCTS

Essential oil blends should always be diluted before application to the skin. Below are guidelines for dilution percentages for various products, from weakest to strongest.

Preparation	Amount of Essential Oil Blend	Amount of Carrier	Percentage Dilution	Notes
Body mists, facial toners	5–10 drops	2 fluid ounces distilled water	1/2–1%	Shake well before use; be sure to close eyes
Room sprays	10–15 drops	2 fluid ounces distilled water	1%	Shake well before use; do not spray on room furniture
Linen, lingerie, clothing, or stationery sprays	20–30 drops	2 fluid ounces distilled water	2%	Shake well; test for staining on hidden area of fabric
Massage, bath, facial, and body oils	5–12 drops	1 fluid ounce vegetable or jojoba oil	1–2%	Use a very weak dilution of only floral oils for children, pregnant women, the elderly, or ill.
Eau de toilette	4–8 drops	92–96 drops of a blend of 1/3 alcohol and 2-3 water	4–8%	Use Everclear, not vodka. Can be applied more generously than perfume.
Perfume	15–30 drops	70–85 drops of pure grain alcohol or jojoba oil	15–30%	Use Everclear, not vodka, for the alcohol. Apply sparingly.

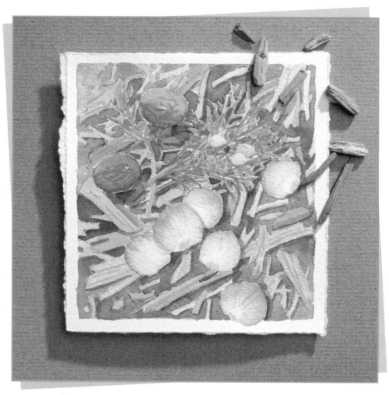

"As other spirits are borne
away on music, mine, my beloved!
floats on your perfume."

— Charles Baudelaire

Forty Fragrant Oils

A professional perfumer may have hundreds of aromatic substances from which to choose. It is possible, however, to create beautiful, unique fragrance blends with as few as two essential oils. In fact, it is often better to keep your first experiments simple.

Following is a list of forty essential oils to use in building your own perfume "organ." Included are the plant source's Latin name; an odor intensity rating; a description of the essential oil's scent; whether it functions as a base, middle, or top note; and suggested blending partners. Brief descriptions detail the reputed therapeutic applications of each oil for physical or emotional conditions. Finally, I've compiled a few informational tidbits about each essential oil. Known circumstances under which these fragrances should *not* be used are also listed.

All essential oils in this list are extracted by distillation, with the exception of jasmine and vanilla, which are absolutes made by solvent extraction. For the recipes containing rose essential oil, either rose otto (distilled rose oil) or rose absolute may be used.

Ambrette

HIBISCUS ABELMOSCHUS

Scent: Sweet, musky, tenacious
Middle to top note
Odor Intensity: 3
Blending companions: Florals, woods, spices
Physical uses: Soothes indigestion, nervous stomach, anxiety, stress, and muscle aches; aphrodisiac
Emotional uses: Depression, negative viewpoint, nervousness
Tidbits: This herb is also known as muskmallow; it functions as a botanical alternative for animal-derived musk fragrance. Ambrette often graces "oriental" fragrances.

Angelica

ANGELICA ARCHANGELICA

Scent: Herbaceous, earthy, peppery, green, spicy
Middle to top note
Odor Intensity: 4

Blending companions: Florals, woods, oriental blends

Physical uses: Respiratory, digestive and reproductive tonic; aphrodisiac, antispasmodic

Emotional uses: Depression, disconnection from higher purpose

Tidbits: A good substitute for ambrette, which can be hard to find. May be distilled from the seeds or the root. Candied angelica stems were a popular European dessert condiment in the Victorian era.

Caution: This plant contains coumarins, which are photosensitizing. If your blend contains this oil, wear it on skin that is protected from the sun.

Basil

OCIMUM BASILICUM

Scent: Herbaceous, spicy, anise-like, camphorous, lively

Middle to top note

Odor intensity: 4

Blending companions: Lavender, rosemary, grapefruit, woods

Physical uses: Stimulant, digestive, anti-spasmodic

Emotional uses: To sharpen the senses, stimulate mental capacity, overcome indecision, improve mental outlook, attract money

Tidbits: From this herbaceous culinary herb comes the delectable Italian dish pesto. Basil's name means "royal," and it is considered sacred in India. There are many chemotypes, or chemical varieties, of this essential oil. The hundreds of cultivars can range in fragrance from cinnamon-spicy to geranium-like, from sharp to lemony.

Caution: Depending on the chemotype, this oil can be irritating to the skin. Do a patch test of any products first.

Bay

LAURUS NOBILIS

Scent: Sweet, fresh, spicy, camphorous, medicinal

Middle to top note

Odor intensity: 3

Blending companions: Rosemary, fir, juniper, lavender, citrus, spices

Physical uses: Lymphatic cleanser, mildly stimulating, antiseptic, sedative

Emotional uses: Psychic shield and protector against negativity; improves intuition, clarity, and perspective

Tidbits: Laurel leaves were woven into

wreaths worn on the heads of Greek and Roman scholars or victors.

Caution: Do not confuse this true culinary bay with the California bay, *Umbellaria californica,* or the more common East Indian allspice bays, *Pimenta racemosa* or *P. dioica;* all of these are skin irritants.

Bergamot

CITRUS BERGAMIA

Scent: Sweet, lively, citrus, fruity
Top note
Odor intensity: 2
Blending companions: Florals, geranium, coriander
Physical uses: Antiseptic, skin astringent, relaxant, digestive
Emotional uses: Depression, anxiety
Tidbits: Named after the Italian city of Bergamot, this is a classic eau de cologne scent. It is also used to flavor Earl Grey tea.
Caution: Bergamot is perhaps the most photosensitizing of all the citrus oils. However, a bergaptene-free essential oil, which is not photosensitizing, is available. This oil may be labeled "FCF bergamot." The acronym stands for furanocoumarin-free.

Cardamom

ELETTARIA CARDOMOMUM

Scent: Sweet, spicy, balsamic with floral undertones.
Middle note
Odor intensity: 4
Blending companions: Citrus, florals, cedar, frankincense
Physical uses: Antispasmodic, aphrodisiac, digestive, stimulating
Emotional uses: Mental fatigue, anxiety, anorexia, cluttered consciousness
Tidbits: A classic Indian spice and a standard in the tea beverage, chai, cardamom is also used in Latin America, China, Europe, and the Middle East.

Carrot seed

DAUCUS CAROTA

Scent: Sweet, fruity, warm, earthy
Middle note
Odor intensity: 2
Blending companions: Frankincense, geranium, citrus, spices
Physical uses: Digestive tonic, fatigue; mature or sun-damaged skin, rashes
Emotional uses: Revitalizes energy of the solar plexus

Tidbits: This is the common roadside weed Queen Anne's Lace, also known as Bird's Nest Fern because of the way the seed pods fold in a circular pattern like a bird's nest. It is also the ancestor of our common garden carrot. In fact, the Latin name is the same, with only varietal name distinctions.

Cedar, Atlas

CEDRUS ATLANTICA

Scent: Warm, soft, woody
Base note
Odor intensity: 3
Blending companions: Bergamot, florals, resins, clary sage
Physical uses: Relaxing, aphrodisiac, circulatory tonic; eases dandruff and acne
Emotional uses: Assists meditation, self-control, grounding, emotional strength in a crisis, determination
Tidbits: This tree is also known as Lebanon cedar or Himalayan cedar, and was used medicinally in Tibet, as an incense in the East, and as an embalming herb in Egypt. The wood was also treasured as a naturally insect-repellent building material.

Caution: Do not confuse this precious fragrance with the juniper oils, also sold as cedars, or the very toxic Thuja oil, also known as cedar leaf.

Chamomile, German

MATRICARIA RECUTITA

Scent: Deep, rich, tenacious, cocoa-like, herbaceous
Middle note
Odor intensity: 4
Blending companions: Florals, citrus, clary sage, geranium, patchouli.
Physical uses: Sedative, anti-inflammatory; soothes sensitive skin, promotes wound healing
Emotional uses: Eases oversensitivity, tension, hysteria, anxiety; invites emotional support
Tidbits: This is the common tea herb so classic to English children's stories. The presence of azulene, a component produced in the heat of distillation, colors the essential oil a beautiful blue.

Chamomile, Roman

CHAMAEMELUM NOBILE
(ANTHEMIS NOBILIS)

Scent: Fresh, sweet, fruity-herbaceous, apple-like
Middle note
Odor intensity: 4
Blending companions: Florals, citrus, geranium, lavender, patchouli
Physical uses: Anti-spasmodic, relaxing, skin supporting, antiseptic, wound healing
Emotional uses: Tension, depression; times when harmony and self-control are important
Tidbits: This perennial herb was once planted in English lawns to release its wonderfully fruity-floral scent when trod upon. The herb is medicinal, but has a very bitter flavor and is not often used as tea.

Cinnamon

CINNAMOMUM ZEYLANICUM

Scent: Spicy, warm, sweet
Middle note
Odor intensity: 5
Blending companions: Citrus, woods
Physical uses: Stimulating, warming, digestive, antispasmodic
Emotional uses: Energizing, increases feelings of abundance and prosperity, stimulates psychic awareness
Tidbits: This native of the Near and Far East produces essential oil from the leaves (mild) and inner bark (sweet and hot). Cassia oil *(C. cassia)* is similar in fragrance.
Caution: Both cinnamon and cassia essential oils are skin irritants. Use sparingly in any blend.

Clary sage

SALVIA SCLAREA

Scent: Herbaceous, spicy, hay-like; sharp, fixative
Middle to base note
Odor intensity: 3
Blending companions: Lavender, geranium, woods, citrus
Physical uses: Anti-depressant, menstrual tonic, astringent, aphrodisiac
Emotional uses: Confusion, indecision, PMS, postpartum depression, panic and a sense of being overwhelmed
Tidbits: This herb was known in Medieval Europe as "clear eyes." The Latin

species name, sclaria, hints at its use as a tea for clearing the white, or sclera, of the eyes. Like that of its close relative, garden sage, the distilled essential oil has reputed estrogenic effects.

Coriander

CORIANDRUM SATIVUM

Scent: Woody, spicy, sweet
Middle note
Odor intensity: 3
Blending companions: Clary sage, citrus, firs, spices
Physical uses: Digestive, stimulant, anti-spasmodic, , antiseptic
Emotional uses: Improves motivation, mental determination, helps balance joy and stability
Tidbits: This common domestic spice is used all over the world and was found in the tomb of the Egyptian king Ramses II. A good substitute for endangered rosewood oil.

Fir

ABIES BALSAMEA

Scent: Fresh, clean, green, balsamic, coniferous, sweet
Middle note

Odor intensity: 2
Blending companions: Lavender, rosemary, frankincense, cedar, citrus
Physical uses: Respiratory, circulatory and urinary tonic, antiseptic, adrenal stimulant
Emotional uses: Refreshing, mood elevating, increases intuition, fosters contentment and love
Tidbits: The essential oil distilled from the needles is superior to that of the sap, also known as turpentine. The oil is similar in fragrance to pine and spruce oils. There will be slight fragrance fluctuations among the many varieties and species within those genera, including *Abies, Larix, Picea, Pinus,* and *Tsuga.*

Frankincense

BOSWELLIA CARTERII

Scent: Rich, deep, warm, balsamic, sweet with incense-like overtones
Base note
Odor intensity: 3
Blending companions: Citrus, spices, sandalwood, geranium, lavender, fir
Physical uses: Antiseptic, skin aging, wound healing, expectorant
Emotional uses: Meditative, enhances

spirituality, builds courage, focus, concentration, awareness, insight

Tidbits: This resin's history dates back to antiquity as the "true incense," which is also the translation of its name. Used in ancient India, Egypt, and China, it is still employed in the Catholic church, where it was originally used as both fumigant and sacred scent.

Geranium

PELARGONIUM GRAVEOLENS

Scent: Sweet, green, citrus-rosy, fresh
Middle note
Odor intensity: 3
Blending companions: Florals, citrus, sandalwood, patchouli
Physical uses: Anti-inflammatory, anti-fungal, deodorant, adrenal tonic; skin care
Emotional uses: Stress, discontent; helps improve mental outlook, good for the workaholic who needs to reconnect with the self and emotions
Tidbits: This small flowering, fragrant foliage plant should not be confused with the true genus, *Geranium*, the common window–box plants with the large red blossoms. There are

many varieties of pelargoniums, including *P. asperum* and *P. fragrantissimum*.

Ginger

ZINGIBER OFFICINALE

Scent: Sweet, spicy-woody, warm, tenacious, fresh, sharp
Middle note
Odor intensity: 4
Blending companions: Florals, woods, spices
Physical uses: Digestive tonic, anti-spasmodic, muscle pain, warming stimulant for cold and damp conditions
Emotional uses: Underconfidence, procrastination, lack of vitality or initiative
Tidbits: Known the world over for its culinary and medicinal qualities, ginger grows in tropical climates and is extracted by distillation or carbon dioxide extraction.

Grapefruit

CITRUS ×PARADISI

Scent: Clean, fresh, bitter, citrusy
Top note
Odor intensity: 2
Blending companions: Citrus, lavender,

geranium, neroli, jasmine, carrot seed

Physical uses: Oily skin problems, cellulite, lymphatic drainage, depression, fatigue

Emotional uses: Uplifting; good for performance anxiety, self-critcism, guilt, anger, frustration

Tidbits: Oils extracted by cold expression have a superior fragrance, but those produced by distillation have fewer of the photosensitizing coumarins, making them safer for use with sun exposure.

Caution: Photosensitizing

Helichrysum

HELICHRYSUM ANGUSTIFOLIA
VAR. ITALICUM

Scent: Rich, sweet, fruity with tea and honey undertones

Middle note

Odor intensity: 3

Blending companions: Geranium, clary sage, rose, lavender, spices, citrus

Physical uses: Good for mature skin, arthritis, inflammation, bruising, muscle strain; antispasmodic

Emotional uses: Drug detoxification; addictive and judgmental behavior, self-denial, bitterness; fosters creativity and feelings of compassion

Tidbits: This common garden shrub is called curry plant, owing to its spicy scent, and it resembles a santolina. Its gray-green foliage produces small yellow blossoms that retain their shape and color upon drying.

Jasmine

JASMINUM OFFICINALE

Scent: Powerful, sweet, tenacious, floral with fruity-herbaceous undertones

Base note

Odor intensity: 4

Blending companions: Citrus, rose, sandalwood, clary sage

Physical uses: Sedative, euphoric, antispasmodic, aphrodisiac

Emotional uses: Good for anger, worry, apathy, lack of confidence; restores creativity, reawakens passion

Tidbits: If rose is Queen of the flowers, then jasmine must surely be King. Solvent extraction of many species, including *J. grandiflorum* and *J. sambac,* yields the absolutes that form the base of so many expensive perfumes. This Asian native has been used to flavor teas and employed in both internal and external medicines.

Juniper

JUNIPERUS COMMUNIS

Scent: Sweet, musky, tenacious
Middle note
Odor intensity: 3
Blending companions: Lavender, rosemary, woods, spices
Physical uses: Helps oily skin and acne; stimulating tonic and diuretic; antirheumatic; helps drive out cold and damp conditions
Emotional uses: Good for mental stagnation, fear of failure, cleansing the emotional environment, releasing past worries, overcoming obstacles, and improving psychological outlook
Tidbits: Juniper oil is distilled from the berries (best) or the branches. There are about sixty species in this genus which was used as an ancient incense herb by many cultures including Native American. It is one of the herbs used in making gin.

Lavender

LAVANDULA ANGUSTIFOLIA

Scent: Floral, sweet, herbaceous, balsamic, woody undertones
Middle note
Odor intensity: 2
Blending companions: Florals, citrus, clary sage, vetiver, patchouli, fir
Physical uses: Wound and burn healing, relaxing, insect bites, anti-inflammatory, all skin care, muscle aches, headache, insomnia
Emotional uses: Releases bad habits, unexpressed emotion, depression; good for manifesting creative potential, for the introverted and inhibited
Tidbits: Many species of this classically floral scent are distilled for use in soaps and perfumes. The camphorous "spike" lavender (*L. latifolia*) is useful for acne skin problems and stiff joints. Another species, lavandin, (*L. ×intermedia)* is a cross between true and spike lavenders. It produces a higher yield of essential oil and is often used to adulterate true lavender oil. Its smell is similar, but it contains only sixty chemical constituents while true lavender has about 160.

Lemon

CITRUS LIMON

Scent: *Sweet, sharp, clear, citrusy*
Top note

Odor intensity: 2
Blending companions: Florals, basil, geranium, frankincense
Physical uses: Digestive, antiviral, anti-rheumatic, liver tonic; decongestant, good for damp heat
Emotional uses: Cleansing, revitalizing, purifying; helps maintain poise and objectivity. Encourages trust, clears intellect, eases confusion
Tidbits: Nutritious and medicinal, lemon oil it was once considered by some to be a cure-all and was used to perfume clothing, cleanse the blood, and repel insects.
Caution: Photosensitizing

Lemongrass

CYMBOPOGON CITRATUS

Scent: Grassy, lemony, pungent, bitter
Top note
Odor intensity: 4
Blending companions: Lavender, jasmine, geranium, clary sage
Physical uses: Astringent, antiseptic, sedative, acne treatment, insect repellent
Emotional uses: Uplifting, awakens psychic and logical skills, fosters new ideas
Tidbits: Just like as name suggests, this oil is distilled from the leaves of the lemony-scented grass. It is native to Asia and now grows in many tropical regions, where it is enjoyed in refreshing beverages.
Caution: Skin irritant; use sparingly.

Lime

CITRUS AURANTIIFOLIA

Scent: Sweet, tart, intense, lively
Top note
Odor intensity: 3
Blending companions: Florals, woods, spices
Physical uses: Stimulating, cleansing, digestive, anti-viral, general tonic; good for oily skin
Emotional uses: Mental and emotional clearing; helps in creating emotional space and independence, moves one to action
Tidbits: Lime essential oil may be expressed or distilled; the expression process yields a fresh fragrance while distillation yields one that is candy-like. Don't confuse lime oil with that of lime blossom, *Tillia europaea,* more frequently called linden.
Caution: Expressed oil is photosensitizing; distilled is not.

Marjoram

ORIGANUM MAJORANA
(MAJORANA HORTENSIS)

Scent: Herbaceous, green, spicy
Middle note
Odor intensity: 3
Blending companions: Lavender, rosemary, bergamot, juniper, geranium
Physical uses: Anti-inflammatory, antispasmodic, muscle relaxant, respiratory tonic, sedative
Emotional uses: Despair, despondency and self-pity; fosters self-nurturing, honoring; comforting, restores hope
Tidbits: This plant's family name of oregano is from the Greek *oros* and *ganos,* meaning "joy of the mountain." Marjoram was historically believed to bring spiritual peace to the dead. This is "sweet" marjoram; do not confuse it with "wild" or "Spanish" marjoram (*Thymus mastachina*).

Neroli

CITRUS ARANTIUM
VAR. AMARA OR C. BIGARADIA

Scent: Floral, citrusy, sweet, delicate, slightly bitter
Middle note
Odor intensity: 3
Blending companions: Blends well with all oils, especially florals
Physical uses: Calming, anti-depressant; good for mature skin, broken capillaries, and other skin problems
Emotional uses: For anxiety, emotional shock, fear of public speaking, fatigue, lack of confidence; also to promote emotional harmony, release deep pain, and encourage hope
Tidbits: This species of citrus fruit produces three different essential oils from one plant: neroli from the blossom, bitter orange from the peel, and petitgrain from the leaves. The tree is native to Italy and is named after the princess of Nerola. It was traditionally used in bridal bouquets to calm the nerves of newlyweds.

Nutmeg

MYRISTICA FRAGRANS

Scent: Sweet, musky, spicy
Middle note
Odor intensity: 4
Blending companions: Florals, woods, spices
Physical uses: Digestive tonic, antiseptic; for nervous fatigue, impotence

Emotional uses: To boost optimism about money and luck, overcome confusion and fatigue

Tidbits: Nutmeg is produced by the same tropical tree as mace; the latter is the lacy covering that surrounds the seed. Europeans in the seventeenth century often carried nutmeg and tiny graters to flavor food and drinks.

Caution: Overuse of this essential oil can cause headaches, confusion, and hypnotic dreams.

Orange

CITRUS SINENSIS

Scent: Fresh, citrusy, fruity, sweet, light

Top note

Odor intensity: 1

Blending companions: Florals, spices, clary sage, frankincense

Physical uses: Anti-depressant, sedative, antiseptic, stimulant

Emotional uses: Uplifting to the spirit, increases tolerance, compassion, and joy; to disperses moodiness

Tidbits: This native of the Far East is extracted by cold expression. Its lively scent is one of the most recognized and utilized of all essential oils.

Caution: Photosensitizing

Palmarosa

CYMBOPOGON MARTINI

Scent: Lemony, fresh, green, with hints of rose and geranium

Middle to top notes

Odor intensity: 3

Blending companions: Ylang ylang, lavender, geranium, coriander, florals, woods

Physical uses: For acne and psoriasis; relaxant, analgesic, antibacterial; genito-urinary tonic

Emotional uses: To encourage emotional flexibility and personal security; to comfort the heart, clear grief, relieve clingyness and possessiveness

Tidbits: Distilled since the 1700s, this member of the grass family is related to lemongrass and citronella. It is cooling in nature, and was once used to adulterate rose oil. It shares with geranium the fragrant component geraniol.

Patchouli

POGOSTEMON CABLIN

Scent: Earthy, herbaceous, sweet-balsamic, rich, with woody undertones

Base note

Odor intensity: 4

Blending companions: Frankincense, clary sage, lavender, geranium, sandalwood, rose, citrus

Physical uses: Anti-inflammatory, wound healing, anti-depressant; for mature skin care

Emotional uses: For meditation, sexual arousal, manifesting desired wealth; to quiet mental overactivity

Tidbits: When shawls from India were sold in England without the signature odor of patchouli, used to deter bugs, sales lagged. The essential oil is distilled from the dried and fermented leaves and is even used to flavor soft drinks.

Pepper

PIPER NIGRUM

Scent: Spicy, peppery, musky, warm with herbaceous undertones

Middle note

Odor intensity: 3

Blending companions: Lavender, frankincense, rosemary, florals, woods, spices

Physical uses: Warming, digestive, circulatory stimulant, antispasmodic, antiseptic

Emotional uses: To develop mental alertness, enhance stamina for mentally and emotionally draining situations; to remove energy blockages and boost courage; to promote mental and emotional drive

Tidbits: Black pepper is the unripe peppercorn; white pepper is the ripe fruit with the outer pericarp removed.

Peppermint

MENTHA × PIPERITA

Scent: Minty, sharp, intense

Middle note

Odor intensity: 5

Blending companions: Resins, citrus, rosemary, lavender

Physical uses: As an analgesic, anti-inflammatory, respiratory and digestive tonic; to relieve headaches

Emotional uses: To clear the mind of fatigue, promote sharp communication, enhance concentration, develop emotional tolerance

Tidbits: The name *Menthe* comes from the Latin *mente*, meaning thought. Remains of this medicinal herb were found in an Egyptian tomb dating from 1000 B.C. It is said to be an ingredient of the ancient incense *kyphi*.

Mint can have both heating and cooling effects.

Rose

ROSA DAMASCENA

Scent: Floral, spicy, rich, deep, sensual, green, honey-like
Middle to base note
Odor intensity: 3
Blending companions: All oils
Physical uses: Reproductive tonic, PMS, infertility, all skin care, insomnia, anti-depressant, nervous tension, aphrodisiac
Emotional uses: To uplift the spirit, transform sexual love to spiritual connection, develop tolerance; heal emotional wounds, especially heartache; banish envy, jealousy
Tidbits: The queen of all flowers, and the most revered for inspiring spiritual devotion, rose represents love on all levels. Safe and non-toxic, yet a powerful antiseptic and antiviral, rose has a history of use throughout civilization and a multitude of cultures as a food, medicine, and cosmetic. The distillation of *R. damascena* produces rose otto, a middle note. The solvent extraction of *R. centifolia* produces rose absolute, more often categorized as a base note.

Rosemary

ROSMARINUS OFFICINALIS

Scent: Herbaceous, strong, camphorous, with woody-balsamic and evergreen undertones
Middle note
Odor intensity: 3
Blending companions: Cedar, frankincense, lavender, geranium, citrus
Physical uses: Stimulant, antioxidant; liver, circulatory and respiratory tonic; muscle aches; hair care
Emotional uses: Remembrance, invigoration; to boost low self-esteem, to manifest love and increase faith in one's potential
Tidbits: The name means "dew of the sea." Legend has it that the Virgin Mary stopped to rest near a large rosemary plant; after she had laid her cloak upon the shrub, all the flowers turned from white to blue. Rosemary has always been known as an herb of medicine, food, and magic, and a protector against evil.

Sandalwood

SANTALUM ALBUM

Scent: Soft, woody, sweet, earthy, balsamic, tenacious

Base note

Odor intensity: 3

Blending companions: Florals, spices, geranium, vetiver, patchouli, coriander

Physical uses: Sedative, genito-urinary and respiratory tonic; soothes dry skin

Emotional uses: To uplift spirit and psyche; for grounding and meditation; to ease obsessive worry and attachment; for the intellectually over-driven

Tidbits: The sandalwood tree takes forty years to develop its fragrance, which is distilled from the center heartwood. Revered as sacred, this wood was used to build temples. Its scent lulled worshippers into a state of devotional bliss while the essential oil acted as a natural insecticide to deter a multitude of tropical bugs from disrupting services.

Spikenard

NARDOSTACHYS JATAMANSI

Scent: Heavy, earthy, animal-like, similar to valerian

Base note

Odor intensity: 5

Blending companions: Lavender, fir, spices, citrus

Physical uses: Nervous indigestion and insomnia, stress, aging skin, psoriasis, allergies

Emotional uses: To soothe anxiety, despondency, depression, and resentment; encourage compassion and acceptance; as a sacred and ancient anointing oil

Tidbits: Known to the Egyptians, Romans, and the Greek physician Dioscorides, this sacred plant was mentioned in the Song of Solomon in the Bible; its oil was used by Mary Magdalene to anoint the feet of Jesus Christ.

Vanilla

VANILLA PLANIFOLIA

Scent: Sweet, balsamic, heavy, warm

Base note

Odor intensity: 4

Blending companions: Florals, woods, citrus, spices

Physical uses: Sedative, antidepressant

Emotional uses: To convey comfort, nurturing, security; foster maternal instinct, build confidence, soften frustration and anger

Tidbits: Vanilla is the only edible orchid in the world. It is native to Central America where its only natural pollinator, the melipone bee, is found. It is now grown in Tahiti, Madagascar, and Indonesia, where its cultivators rely on hand pollination. A comforting scent for children.

Vetiver

VETIVERIA ZIZANOIDES

Scent: Heavy, earthy, balsamic, smoky, sweet undertones
Base note
Odor intensity: 5
Blending companions: Woods, spices, resins, florals, clary sage
Physical uses: Wound healing, acne and oily skin, muscle pain, insomnia, sprains
Emotional uses: Sedating yet restorative; to soothe a hyperactive mind, reconnect to the inner self
Tidbits: The vetiver plant is a grass, but the essential oil is distilled from its thin, hair-like roots.

Ylang ylang

CANANGA ODORATA
VAR. GENUINA

Scent: Sweet, heavy, narcotic, cloying, tropical floral, with spicy-balsamic undertones
Middle to base note
Odor intensity: 5
Blending companions: Clary sage, vetiver, floral, citrus, woods
Physical uses: Anti-depressant, sedative, hypertension, aphrodisiac; for oily skin
Emotional uses: Nervousness, euphoria; to transform negative and stagnant emotional states; to open, center, and unify the spirit
Tidbits: This tropical flower is so sweet, it almost smells synthetic. Its distillation produces four grades of oil: ylang "extra," considered the highest grade, and subsequent distillations graded one, two, and three. A still lower quality oil, known as Cananga, is produced from *Cananga odorata var. Macrophylla.*

ESSENTIAL OILS: NOTE TYPE AND ODOR INTENSITY

This chart lists the odor intensity of top, middle, and base notes in order of odor intensity, with 1 being the lightest and 5 the strongest.

ESSENTIAL OIL	ODOR INTENSITY
Top Notes	
Orange	1
Lemon	2
Bergamot	2
Grapefruit	2
Lime	3
Lemongrass	4
Middle to Top Notes	
Ambrette	3
Bay	3
Palmarosa	3
Angelica	4
Basil	4
Middle Notes	
Carrot seed	2
Fir	2
Lavender	2
Coriander	3
Geranium	3
Helichrysum	3
Juniper	3
Marjoram	3
Neroli	3
Chamomile, German	4

ESSENTIAL OIL	ODOR INTENSITY
Middle Notes (continued)	
Pepper	3
Rosemary	3
Cardamom	4
Chamomile, Roman	4
Ginger	4
Nutmeg	4
Peppermint	5
Cinnamon	5
Middle to Base Notes	
Clary sage	3
Rose	3
Ylang ylang	5
Base Notes	
Cedar, Atlas	3
Frankincense	3
Sandalwood	3
Jasmine	4
Patchouli	4
Vanilla	4
Spikenard	5
Vetiver	5

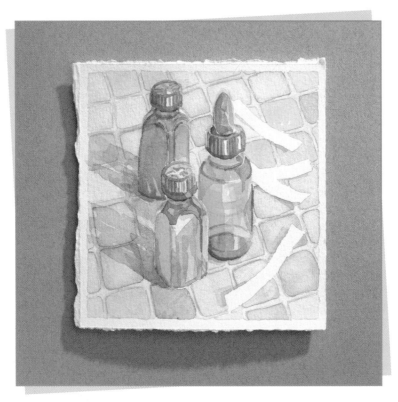

"I have loved flowers that fade,
  within whose magic tents
rich hues have marriage made
with sweet unmemoried scents."

— Robert Bridges

Two Beginning Blending Lessons

*C*reative perfumery is about inspiration. Listen to your intuition, throw out all the rules (except those of safety), and develop an adventurous attitude. Your inspiration for a particular perfume may arrive via an event or poem that moves you emotionally, a holiday that brings joy, or an appreciation of a bit of nature such as a waterfall or a wildflower meadow. Whatever it is, indulge your passion, be bold, unencumbered, and enjoy the endeavor. In other words, have fun!

My suggestion is that you first try to create a scent that captures an aspect of your personality. Explore your character for clues to what fragrance blends you like. If you are a hopeless romantic, you may be attracted to the poetic odors of florals, balanced with a hint of green and a slight, softly woody note. If you are outgoing and athletic, you may be drawn to a more exhilarating scent that energizes, with a citrus top note, a splash of spicy/green, and a hint of clear woods or crisp fir. If you are shy and understated, you may prefer single, uncomplicated scents or simple florals with a hint of fruit to reflect your innocence. Sexy and sultry types will likely choose to indulge in mysterious, tenacious, and devoted base notes, with a hint of inviting and seductive florals. If you are assured and refined, you may favor scents that sparkle and contribute to your confidence, such as a brilliant combination of floral and citrus bouquets. Whatever route you take, let your intuition guide you.

LESSON 1: PLAYING WITH SCENT CLASSIFICATIONS

Throughout classical perfumery, several masters have created themes on which to base their fragrance blends. Some perfume artists composed a scent as one would a symphony, associating fragrance notes with those on a musical scale. Others classified odors on a numerical basis. Some found the metaphor of painting the most apt; they blended odors as an artist blends colors.

All categorizations of fragrance are in some ways artificial and arbitrary. Nonetheless, they may help you find ways to characterize the scents you'll be blending. For your first outing as a perfumer, I've guided you through the categories below, which adapt well to natural ingredients and the forty oils listed in this book. Call it a little nose exercise. The essential oils that fall into these categories have some similar qualities; to achieve the effect of that category, you may need to include only one or two in your blend. Sometimes using a small quantity of each will do the trick. If budget is a factor, choose just a few of these scent categories that you find attractive.

As you play and enjoy, share your experiments with a few friends, take notes, or run a small tape recorder. Notice what you like and dislike. You may discover a blend that you'll enjoy for a lifetime, or the perfect expression of a friend's true beauty.

ANISIC
Licorice-like: Anise, fennel, basil

Fragrances in this category have a high odor intensity. They mix well with citrus oils or woods, each creating a very different fragrance.

Try, on two separate strips of blotter paper, one drop each of anise and basil. Add a few drops of lemon to each to give the scents some lift. Experience the scent for a while; note the differences. Now try adding one or two drops of geranium or lavender for a bit of a floral note.

BALSAMIC
Sweet, warm, soft, earthy odors: Vetiver, sandalwood, cedar

These are among my favorite scents. Since sandalwood and cedar have a lower odor intensity than vetiver, we will use more of them. In a small, clean glass bottle, blend three drops sandalwood, two drops cedar, and one drop vetiver. Try this one on the inside of your wrist; be sure to give it an hour or more to fully develop on your skin. This blend can be used alone, or as a base note in another formula.

To see how, dip two strips of blotter paper into your bottle. Add a drop of bergamot to one; for an herbaceous note, add a drop of lavender to the other. Does either one call your name? If one of these scents is almost, but not quite, perfect, you can add more of the balsamic blend, or more of either floral.

CAMPHORACEOUS
Clean, fresh, medicinal: Rosemary, lavender, eucalyptus

These classically clean scents really grab your attention, and are often used in therapeutic blends. They can give your fragrance a sharp edge, if that's the effect you're seeking, and they're good mood modifiers. Try this combination for a blend that will stimulate the senses and open the respiratory tract. In a clean bottle, combine three drops rosemary, two drops lavender, and one drop eucalyptus.

Now, for an earthy quality, add single drop by drop, some vetiver. If a woody note is more to your liking, do the same thing with cedar instead.

CITRUS
Uplifting, fresh, cool, clear: Bergamot, orange, lime, lemongrass, grapefruit

These top notes are sharp and invigorating. Like a prelude to a fragrance, they will make you want to stop, inhale deeply, and take in their sweet, fruity notes. Within this group of oils, lemongrass has the highest odor intensity.

Begin blending with four drops bergamot, three drops orange, two drops grapefruit, and one drop lemongrass. Test this blend; Are there fragrance notes that you want to accentuate? If so, try adding one more drop of them. Test again.

This blend can be used as a top note in other blends; it works well with florals. Try some jasmine for a heady, aphrodisiacal scent. Add it single drop by drop, testing all the while. Or, to take the blend in a sweet-oriental direction, add a drop each of vanilla and sandalwood. These notes are popular in aftershave ingredients.

FLORAL
Fresh, spring-like, sometimes herbaceous: Rose, jasmine, ylang ylang

Sweet, euphoric, aphrodisiac, and heady, these fragrances are often expensive. They serve well as accentuators in a blend. If used properly they won't overpower the fragrance, but make it stronger, more itself. For a signature feminine fragrance, they can be used alone. Try three drops rose, two drops jasmine, and only one drop ylang ylang, as this last oil is almost narcotic in its sweetness.

Ready to play some more? Try lemon oil, drop by drop, to keep the blend light, but add freshness. Want a rich, exotic note instead? Add frankincense or sandalwood, again, drop by drop.

FORESTLIKE
Wet, mossy, woodsy scents:
Fir, pine, spruce

These clean smells invite deep breathing. Trees function as the lungs of the earth, giving us more oxygen than any other plant. Coniferous scents are good for the respiratory system and will provide a clean, fresh note to any blend.

In a clean bottle, start with three drops spruce, two drops pine, and one drop fir. Because all these oils have the same odor intensity, they can also be used in equal parts. Or, if one of them particularly pleases you, bump that amount up by a drop.

Now, for step two—To create a grounding, yet uplifting scent, add one of the woody oils—vetiver, sandalwood, or cedar. To produce a classic, sporty fra-grance for a man, add any of the citrus oils, or one drop of the citrus blend.

GREEN
Fresh, light, and grassy: Lavender,
chamomile, geranium

Like new-mown hay, these fragrances provide a leafy, green, or grassy note to your blend. It is almost impossible to go wrong with these three scents together. Blend three drops lavender, two drops geranium, and one drop of either Roman or German chamomile. You'll be relaxed in moments.

Want something a little perkier? Add any of the citrus oils — bergamot, orange, lemon, lime, grapefruit, or lemongrass. To add invigoration and warmth, pick one of the spicy scents: cinnamon, clove, cardamom, ginger, or nutmeg. Again, proceed drop by drop. When it's perfect, you'll know.

POWDERY
Light, dry, faint: Vanilla, sandalwood

I love the "dry-out" note of these soft scents. These are nice in women's or children's blends; they can help lull small ones to sleep and instill a sense of safety and security in grownups. Try two drops of vanilla and three drops of sandalwood. Very nice!

Now, For a twist: add five drops of orange. This aroma may take you back to childhood Dreamsicles—those vanilla ice cream bars coated with a frozen orange crust.

RESINOUS

Buttery, soft, deep: Frankincense, myrrh, cistus, benzoin

These base notes will add depth to any blend. With a scent reminiscent of butterscotch, they'll lull you to the security of the earth's core where you can rest and rejuvenate in a fetal position. These saps help heal the wounds on the surface of their home plants; aromatherapists believe they also can help heal the skin and wounds of the soul. For a first blend, try three drops of benzoin, two drops of frankincense, and one drop of myrrh. I predict you'll agree: This is a scent one could bestow on royalty. It's a wonderful fragrance for use in spiritual ceremony.

SPICY

Hot, sweet, sharp: Cinnamon, ginger, clove, cardamom, nutmeg, pepper

Be careful with these hot, spicy essential oils. With most of them, a very small quantity goes a long way. You may want to do a patch test to check for skin reactions if they are included in a blend; you may also want to dilute them in jojoba oil before testing them on your own skin.

These scents are popular in men's colognes, and as accents in blends that need an edge or in holiday products. To experiment, blend one drop each of the first five oils. It's almost like pumpkin pie!

LESSON 2: SEVENTEEN BASIC BLENDS

Now that you've taken an olfactory tour through some scent categories, let's develop fragrances that will create memories. Natural perfumery need not be complicated. Nature has created depth and dimension within single oils, making it easy to create a complete, complex perfume with only a few ingredients. To give yourself some confidence, you may wish to start simply, and since some essential oils are costly, you'll only need a few of the ones listed in this book to make a pleasing scent. Here are seventeen natural oil combinations that make uncomplicated, yet pleasing fragrances.

Start with three drops of the first oil, two of the second and one of the third.

From there, build the scent to please your sensibilities. Remember to keep notes on how the scent progresses as you blend in each additional drop. These combinations will demonstrate clearly how the high odor-intensity oils can overwhelm a blend. For instance, in the first blend, you may find the cardamom overwhelming even though you use only one drop. You can add more orange and notice how the scent's personality changes. Keep in mind that essential oils of the same plant, but from different suppliers, different years, or different areas of the globe may differ in fragrance and intensity.

You may need to adjust the proportions of a recipe slightly to achieve an effect that you enjoy. With the second foresty blend, for example, the fir will dominate. If you want a woodsier note, add more of the cedar. The third blend is made up of oils that all have a high odor intensity. Which odor do you want to be dominant—sweet ylang ylang, musty patchouli, or green, citrusy lemongrass? The fifth combination is a simple start for an oriental fragrance; a little patchouli or sandalwood would soften it; cinnamon would spice it up. The next two both have vanilla, but they are oh, so different.

You get the idea. Now you are on your way—happy blending!

1. **Orange, German chamomile, cardamom**

2. **Fir, orange, cedar**

3. **Lemongrass, patchouli, ylang ylang**

4. **Grapefruit, lavender, geranium**

5. **Frankincense, fir, orange**

6. **Bergamot, vanilla, angelica**

7. **Sandalwood, lavender, vanilla**

8. **Bergamot, carrot, jasmine**

9. **Fir, rosemary, bergamot**

10. **Neroli, geranium, Roman chamomile**

11. **Sandalwood, ambrette, vetiver**

12. **Rose, geranium, helichrysum**

13. **Lavender, clary sage, marjoram**

14. **Frankincense, lavender, jasmine**

15. **Coriander, orange, spikenard**

16. **Rosemary, cedar, palmarosa**

17. **Bergamot, sandalwood, clary sage**

Thirty Natural Fragrance Recipes

*n*ow that you have a little more experience and an understanding of the principles of blending, here are a few slightly more complex ideas to stimulate your imagination. Feel free to go from melody to improvisation, orchestrating your own personal symphony of fragrance. The oils in these formulations are given by number of drops, but you can scale them up to milliliters as long as the same proportions are retained. The recipes are decidedly minute, due to the price of the oils and the necessity for diluting them before use. Doubling a recipe can require a bit of adjustment. For instance, you may not need to double those oils with high odor intensity. Let your nose be your guide.

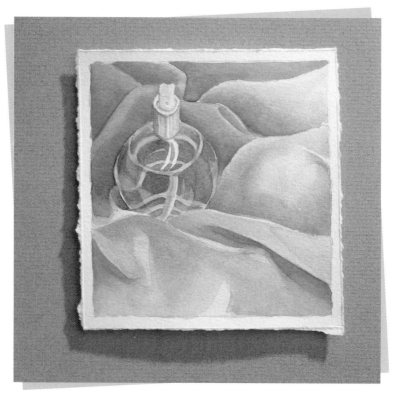

"*There are perfumes as fresh as the
skin of children, gentle as
the oboe, green as the prairie, and
others that are debauched, rich
and triumphant.*"

— *Charles Baudelaire*

These first two scents come from a class I taught for Valentine's Day. They are simple, yet get the message across. Their floral and seductive qualities are wonderful in mists for body or bed linens.

Don't Be Shy

12 drops orange

8 drops sandalwood

5 drops rose

2 drops neroli

Wild About You

18 drops grapefruit

6 drops jasmine

3 drops carrot

1 drop ambrette

Rose Essence

An inexpensive rose perfume with soft undertones. Add this blend to one ounce of grain alcohol and three ounces of distilled water for a refreshing body splash.

6 drops rose

4 drops geranium

3 drops sandalwood

2 drops lemon

1 drop coriander

Heart Guard

Nursing a broken heart? This is just the thing for a comforting scent with a bit of psychic protection. Add this to your after-bath oil to allay anxiety.

8 drops orange

4 drops rose

1 drop ylang ylang

1 drop spikenard

1 drop Roman chamomile

Lullaby

This is a perfect blend for fussiness at any age. Add five to eight drops to a bath for an adult. Mix two drops in one teaspoon vegetable oil for a child's bath.

8 drops lavender

4 drops orange

3 drops neroli

2 drops Roman chamomile

2 drops sandalwood

Simple Delight

This clean blend combines several scent categories. It's sweet, earthy, and floral.

15 drops orange

6 drops frankincense

2 drops atlas cedar

2 drops jasmine

These next two perfume blends are suitable for first fragrances for an adolescent girl. The first is warm and magical, the second fresh and sassy.

Sugar and Spice

10 drops FCF bergamot
(For more on FCF bergamot, see page 33)

5 drops geranium

2 drops vanilla

1 drop Roman chamomile

1 drop cardamom

Everything Nice

8 drops lavender

5 drops grapefruit

3 drops orange

1 drop ylang ylang

1 drop cinnamon leaf

Angel's Whisper

This blend is smooth, sweet, and delicate. The dry-out note lingers, soft and haunting.

4 drops orange

2 drops angelica

2 drops jasmine

1 drop vetiver

1 drop patchouli

Vanilla Caramel Spice

Sweet and dreamy, extra creamy; the name of this concoction says it all. He may just want to gobble you up.

10 drops orange

5 drops vanilla

2 drops vetiver

1 drop cinnamon leaf

1 drop cardamom

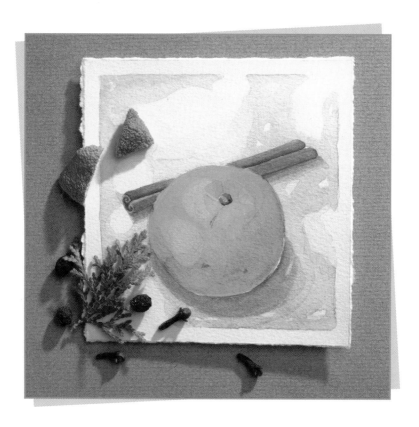

Yuletide Spirit Mist

This blend of essences enhances the holiday spirit and makes a wonderful room mist. You can mix it into a spritz and spray the Christmas tree to keep that fresh, evergreen scent throughout the holiday weeks (not to mention helping keep your tree moist).

15 drops fir

10 drops orange

4 drops frankincense

3 drops bay laurel

3 drops rosemary

2 drops atlas cedar

2 drops vanilla

1 drop peppermint

1 drop cinnamon

Indochine

This scent carries sultry, smoky whiffs of the Orient. It's popular with both men and women.

15 drops orange

10 drops sandalwood

10 drops vanilla

6 drops coriander

5 drops jasmine

3 drops vetiver

1 drop angelica

Incense Cedar

Ancient and primitive, this uplifting, woodsy scent will connect you to nature, even in the city. It makes a wonderful blend to use in an aromatherapy diffuser.

8 drops coriander

6 drops fir

5 drops atlas cedar

5 drops grapefruit

4 drops frankincense

4 drops rosemary

2 drops lemon

2 drops vetiver

2 drops spikenard

1 drop Roman chamomile

Forest

Breathe in the ancient wisdom of the forest, spicy, brisk, crisp, and clean. Take a whiff for an instant get-away at your desk.

10 drops fir

8 drops orange

4 drops helichrysum

3 drops bay laurel

3 drops sandalwood

2 drops coriander

2 drops juniper

1 drop rose absolute

1 drop atlas cedar

Permission

The name alludes to the ingredients in this blend that have reputed aphrodisiacal qualities. Try this one on your next date—it could ignite some flames of desire!

15 drops bergamot

6 drops rose absolute

5 drops jasmine

4 drops coriander

3 drops vanilla

2 drops patchouli

2 drops frankincense

2 drops vetiver

2 drops helichrysum

2 drops clary sage

1 drop nutmeg

Summer Breeze

This scent is sweet and tropical with a hint of spice. Close your eyes, inhale, and escape to the islands. Pure bliss!

5 drops orange

4 drops lime

4 drops vanilla

2 drops neroli

2 drops ylang ylang

1 drop cardamom

1 drop ginger

Restoration

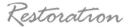

Depressed, dragged out, stressed out, need a little serenity in your life? Five to ten drops of this blend in a relaxing bath and your cares will melt away.

10 drops sandalwood

7 drops bergamot

3 drops clary sage

2 drops ylang ylang

1 drop nutmeg

Egyptian Spice

Enchanting, subtle, unobtrusive, a blend that evokes the hushed silence of an undiscovered temple. Cleopatra had nothing on this!

7 drops coriander

4 drops sandalwood

3 drops lime

3 drops orange

2 drops lavender

2 drops vetiver

1 drop spikenard

1 drop lemongrass

1 drop rosemary

Eau de Cologne

A classic scent, fresh and uplifting. Eau de cologne has always traditionally been made as an alcohol splash. Remember that such alcohol-based scents once doubled as medicine? Indeed, I once used this blend, diluted with grain alcohol and water, as a throat gargle with great success. None of the ingredients is toxic, and the rinse left my mouth freshly clean. To make this oil blend into an alcohol splash, see the blending instructions for eau de toilette on page 29.

8 drops geranium

5 drops neroli

6 drops lavender

5 drops rosemary

4 drops lime

4 drops bergamot

2 drops rose absolute

2 drops petitgrain

2 drops orange

2 drops lemon

2 drops palmarosa

Eau de Fleur

Floral oils make this a joyous blend, suitable diluted as a bath or body oil for a pregnant woman after the first trimester. All the oils are safe and non-toxic; simply add 10 to 15 drops of the blend to two ounces of vegetable oil for a massage oil, or add 5 to 10 drops to a bath. Do not expose skin to sunlight after applying; the bergamot oil is photosensitizing.

7 drops lavender

5 drops bergamot

3 drops rose otto

3 drops neroli

3 drops sandalwood

2 drops jasmine

1 drop Roman chamomile

1 drop ylang ylang

Chocolate Eclipse

The soul yearns for chocolate. It contains phenylethylamine, a chemical produced in the brain when one is in love. You may find this scent a good substitute for a double-fudge brownie.

5 drops German chamomile

5 drops vanilla

2 drops lavender

2 drops orange

2 drops vetiver

1 drop Roman chamomile

1 drop patchouli

Arabian Nights

A fantasy fragrance. This one is attentive, enlightened, aware, regenerating; good at unlocking hidden mysteries. Try it in sesame oil for massages.

4 drops patchouli

4 drops geranium

3 drops frankincense

3 drops rose

3 drops sandalwood

2 drops marjoram

2 drops lemon

2 drops spikenard

1 drop ambrette

China Road

This scent should evoke the journies of Marco Polo, whose daring explorations revealed the sources of many exotic fragrances to the western world.

8 drops frankincense

6 drops marjoram

5 drops sandalwood

2 drops palmarosa

2 drops clary sage

1 drop pepper

1 drop ambrette

1 drop angelica

1 drop ginger

Blue Velvet

Smooth and fresh, yet masculine, aware, and powerful. This blend exudes a presence without being overwhelming.

10 drops sandalwood

5 drops neroli

3 drops carrot

2 drops clary sage

2 drops rosemary

1 drop basil

1 drop lemongrass

1 drop fir

1 drop palmarosa

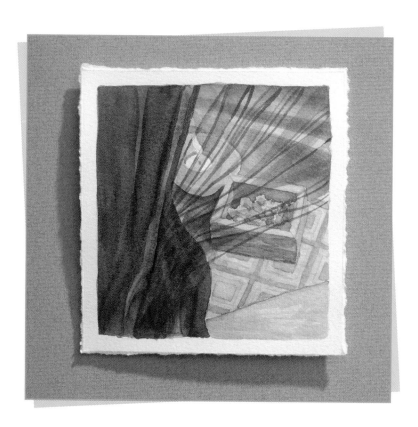

Tantra

Use this scent to awaken your compassion and your open, loving nature. Diluted into a massage oil, the blend is wonderful for sensual massage, and can help lovers evoke a connection on a higher spiritual plane.

10 drops orange

5 drops coriander

5 drops rose

3 drops helichrysum

3 drops lavender

2 drops geranium

2 drops frankincense

1 drop cardamom

Moon Time Balance

I like this combination for easing physical and psychological symptoms of PMS or menopause. Massage this blend, diluted in vegetable oil (see page 29), around the abdomen and hip area, or add eight drops to the bath and soak your troubles away.

10 drops lavender

5 drops geranium

5 drops marjoram

3 drops grapefruit

3 drops clary sage

3 drops rose

1 drop ginger

1 drop ylang ylang

Athena

This is Goddess power: clear, subtle, strong, and secure. A luminous blend of sweet, woodsy, and floral oils to inspire wisdom.

6 drops grapefruit

5 drops rose

4 drops carrot

4 drops sandalwood

2 drops jasmine

2 drops atlas cedar

2 drops rosemary

Lily Milk

This fresh and inspiring blend helps promote a beautiful complexion for any skin type. You can add six to ten drops to an ounce of unscented face or body lotion.

5 drops helichrysum

5 drops lavender

3 drops sandalwood

3 drops neroli

3 drops carrot

3 drops geranium

2 drops Roman chamomile

2 drops jasmine

1 drop palmarosa

1 drop ylang ylang

Amber Unguent

Inspired by the center of the earth and the depths of antiquity: a fragrance that seems to last forever.

9 drops sandalwood

6 drops frankincense

3 drops vanilla

3 drops jasmine

2 drops atlas cedar

2 drops vetiver

2 drops spikenard

1 drop ambrette

1 drop nutmeg

Amber Unguent Perfume Solid

If you want to make this (or any of the other blends) into a solid perfume, warm together a tablespoon of jojoba oil and one-half to one teaspoon of grated beeswax until melted. Allow to cool slightly, but not to the point of solidification; then add one batch of your chosen perfume blend. Let cool until solid.

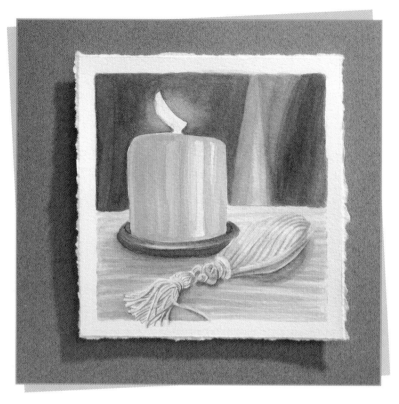

"*Giving a soul to things like poetry,
perfumes know the way of it.*"

— *Guy de Maupassant*

Elemental Blends

ry these elemental blends for ritual work, or for ceremonies celebrating beginnings or endings. Incorporating a special fragrance into an event can provide added power and meaning; years later, smelling the fragrance can bring back memories. Some examples: an anointing ritual at the birth of a child; the cleansing of a new home; celebrating a marriage (or a divorce) and the potential for new beginnings.

There are many occasions when adding scent can inspire or connect us on a deep sensory level, awakening the spirit to the importance of the occasion and endowing the event with special distinction. Try these blends for your rituals, or use them as a beginning to inspire your own unique creations.

Earth
(Meditation)

To help establish and enhance inner strength and establish spiritual and physical grounding; to increase prosperity; to develop patience. Represents the energies of the north.

4 drops cedar

4 drops vanilla

4 drops juniper

2 drops frankincense

2 drops jasmine

2 drops orange

1 drop vetiver

Fire
(Animation)

To help increase strength and the masculine energies; establish power and a warrior spirit; foster sexual balance; break ties with the past; invoke protection and courage. Represents the energies of the south.

6 drops orange

3 drops rosemary

2 drops pepper

1 drop marjoram

1 drop basil

1 drop lime

1 drop cinnamon

Water
(Inspiration)

To help balance the feminine energies; establish a calm emotional balance; increase love, healing, and psychic awareness; invoke spiritual wisdom. Represents the energies of the west.

6 drops geranium

4 drops sandalwood

2 drops German chamomile

2 drops Roman chamomile

2 drops ylang ylang

Air
(Euphoria)

To help stimulate the conscious mind, increase communication and intelligence, and overcome addictions. Represents the energies of the east.

8 drops lavender

4 drops fir

2 drops peppermint

2 drops helichrysum

2 drops clary sage

*"Never think of leaving
perfume or wine to your
heir. Administer these to yourself
and let him have your money."*

— Roman proverb

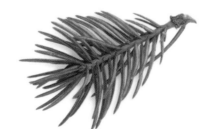

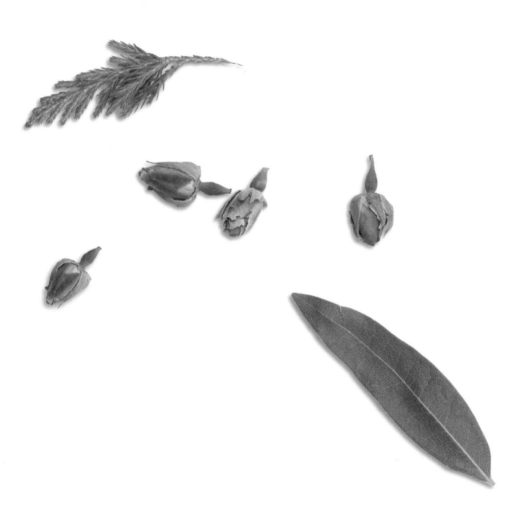

Resource Directory

Many good lines of essential oils can be found in your local health-food store. Here are a few high-quality companies that offer essential oils for purchase by mail-order. Some of them carry unusual oils and rare absolutes.

Amrita Aromatherapy
PO Box 2178
Farifield, IA 52556
(800) 410-9651

Aromatherapy Seminars
117 N. Robertson Blvd.
Los Angeles, CA 90048
(800) 677-2368

Cheryl's Herbs
836 Hanley Industrial Ct.
St. Louis MO 63144
(800) 231-5971
www.cherylsherbs.com

Colin Ingram Company
PO Box 146
Comptche CA 95427
(707) 937-4971
Fax (707) 937-5834
www.coliningram.com

The Essence of Life
7106 NDCBU
Taos, NM 87571
(505) 758-7941
www.taosnet.com/essence

Essential Oil Company
1719 S.E. Umatilla St.
Portland, OR 97202
(800) 729-5912

Fragrant Earth
2000 2nd Ave Suite 206
Seattle, WA 98121
(800) 260-7401
www.fragrantearth.com

Herbal Accents
560 N Coast Hwy. 101 Ste. 4A
Encinitas CA 92024
(760) 633-4255

Leila Castle Botanical Fragrance
PO Box 302
Pt. Reyes Station, CA 94956
(415) 663-1954

Leydet Oils
PO Box 2354
Fair Oaks, CA 95628
(916) 965-7546
www.laydet.com

Lifetime Aromatix
John Steele

3949 Longridge Ave.
Sherman Oaks, CA 91423
(818) 986-0594

Oil Lady Aromatherapy
764 12th Ave. S.
Naples, FL 34102
(941) 263-3451
Fax: (941)263-0898

Original Swiss Aromatics
PO Box 6842
San Rafael, CA 94903
(415) 459-3998
Fax: (415) 479-0119

Primavera Life
1157 Division St.
Napa, CA 94558
(707) 256-0888
(888) 588-9830

Quality of Life
15 Fox Meadow Lane
Deadham, MA 02026
(800) 688-8343

Rainbow Meadow
(800) 207-4047
www.rainbowmeadow.com

Santa Fe Botanical Fragrances Inc.
PO Box 282
Santa Fe, NM 87504
(505) 473-1717
Send SASE for a catalog

Snow Lotus
875 Alpine Ave #5
Boulder, CO 80304
(303) 443-9289

A Women of Uncommon Scents
PO Box 103
Roxbury, PA 17251
(800) 377-3685
(717) 530-0609

PUBLICATIONS

National Association of Holistic Aromatherapists (NAHA)
P.O. Box 17622
Boulder, CO 80308-7622
(888) 275-6242
www.NAHA.org
info@naha.org

American Alliance of Aromatherapy
(quarterly newsletter)
Box 309
Depoe Bay, OR 97341
(800) 809-9850

Aromatic Thymes
(quarterly publication)
18-4 E. Dundee Rd #200
Barrington, IL 60010
(847) 304-0975

Bibliography

Ackerman, Diane. *A Natural History of the Senses.* New York: Vintage Books, 1991.

Cunningham, Scott. *Magical Aromatherapy.* Minnesota: Llewellyn, 1989.

Gloss, R. et al. *The H & R Book of Perfume.* Hamburg, Germany: Verlagsgesellshaft, 1992.

——*Fragrance Guide Feminine Notes.* Hamburg, Germany: Verlagsgesellshaft, 1992.

——*Fragrance Guide Masculine Notes.* Hamburg, Germany: Verlagsgesellshaft, 1992.

——*Guide to Fragrance Ingredients.* Hamburg, Germany: Verlagsgesellshaft, 1992.

Greer, Mary. *The Essence of Magic: Tarot, Ritual, and Aromatherapy.* Van Nuys, California: Newcastle,1993.

Hirsch, Alan, M.D. *Scentsational Sex: The Secret to Using Aroma for Arousal.* Boston, Massachusetts: Element Books, 1998.

Keville, Kathi, and Mindy Green. *Aromatherapy: A Complete Guide to the Healing Art.* Freedom, California: The Crossing Press, 1995.

Lawless, Julia. *The Encyclopedia of Essential Oils.* Rockport, Massachusetts: Element Books, 1992.

LeGuerer, Annick. *Scent: The Mysterious and Essential Powers of Smell.* New York: Turtle Bay Books, 1992.

Miller, Richard Alan. *The Magical & Ritual Use of Perfumes.* New York: Inner Traditions, 1990.

Mojay, Gabriel. *Aromatherapy for Healing the Spirit.* New York: Henry Holt, 1996.

Morris, Edwin T. *Fragrance: The Story of Perfume from Cleopatra to Chanel.* New York: Charles Scribner's, 1984.

Parry, Ernest: *Parry's Cyclopedic of Perfumery.* Vol. I-II. Philadelphia: Blakiston, 1925.

Price, Shirley. *Practical Aromatherapy: How to Use Essential Oils to Restore Vitality.* Wellingborough, England: Thorsons, 1983.

Index

More Herb Books

From Interweave Press

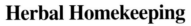

Herbal Homekeeping
Simple Recipes for a Naturally Clean Abode

Sandy Maine

Dozens of chemical-free, earth-friendly recipes to clean everything from laundry and dishes to bathrooms, pets, and leather goods.

Paperback $12.95 U.S./$19.95 Canada plus shipping & handling

Soothing Soaps for Healthy Skin

Sandy Maine

Easy steps for making beautiful, healing soaps. Sandy Maine, author of the Soap Book, collects 24 lye-free recipes.

Paperback $10.95 U.S./$16.95 Canada plus shipping & handling

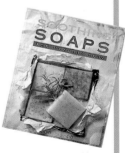

The Herb Tea Book
Blending, Brewing, and Savoring Teas for Every Mood and Occasion

Susan Clotfelter

Blending your own herb tea is not only easy, but healthful, inexpensive, and fun! With 50 recipes.

Paperback $12.95 U.S./$19.95 Canada plus shipping & handling

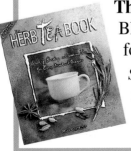